Contents

What Is Sugar Busters Diet?

Sugar Busters! is a low-carb diet and lifestyle book based on the premise that eliminating sugar from the diet will achieve weight loss, fight obesity, and improve overall health

A sugar buster diet plan is a tried and tested method of losing weight without cutting down or marking on the calories. This kind of diet plan includes diet food that is rich with fibre, which helps in better digestion of the consumed food. A sugar busters diet includes fruits, veggies and required nutrition. One exception is to letting go of refined sugar and flour.

This diet became popularized by the 1995 book, "Sugar Busters! Cut Sugar to Trim Fat" by H.

Leighton Steward, Sam S. Andrews, Morrison C. Bethea, and Luis A. Balart. All but Steward are medical doctors

The Sugar Busters eating plan eliminates added sugars, restricts carbohydrates, and emphasizes the consumption of most (but not all) fruits and vegetables, whole grains, lean proteins, low-fat dairy products, and healthy fats. The program is based on consuming foods with a low glycemic index (GI) to maintain optimal blood sugar levels. High GI foods tend to raise blood sugar, which often factors into overeating and weight gain.

Though the diet is relatively balanced and may promote weight loss, it restricts certain healthy foods and lacks scientific evidence. Learn more about the Sugar Busters diet to determine whether this program is the right choice for you.

What You Need to Know

While the rules on the Sugar Busters diet seem fairly straightforward, the program does also allow for some flexibility with the percentages. This could generate confusion around certain foods and how much you should eat in order to meet your goals. For instance, the creators of the program state that you can consume as much as 50–55% of calories from carbs, but they don't offer recommendations for how to adjust your fat and protein intake.

The Sugar Busters diet books don't offer specific measurements for portions, but simply recommend that you consume one plate of food at mealtime and that the plate should not be overly full. Guidelines suggest that you put reasonable portions on the plate and don't go back for seconds.

People on the Sugar Busters diet can consume foods throughout the day according to their preference. They can eat anywhere from three to six meals per day, but the authors advise no eating after 8 p.m. They also suggest that fruits and juices (those that are allowed) should be consumed separately from other foods.

What Can You Eat?

The Sugar Busters diet recommends that about 40% of calories in the diet come from high fiber, low glycemic carbohydrates. In addition, 30% of daily calories should come from lean protein sources like chicken and fish, and about 30–40% of calories from fat (primarily unsaturated fats). Low glycemic index (GI) foods have a value of 55 or less. These foods include most fruits and vegetables, whole grains, some dairy products, and healthy fats like nuts and olive oil.

What to Eat

- Lower-glycemic fruits and vegetables

- Whole grains

- Nuts and legumes

- Lean meats

- Eggs

- Fish and seafood

- Low-fat dairy products

What Not to Eat

- High-glycemic fruits and vegetables

- Refined carbohydrates

- Sugar

- Beer

- Caffeine (in excess)

Lower-Glycemic Fruits and Vegetables

Some fresh, canned, and frozen fruits and vegetables are included in this diet except for the ones listed as high-glycemic. For example, canned fruits should not be packed in syrup. But this is an area where it's easy to get confused about which foods to include and which ones to avoid. For example, sweet potatoes are listed as a compliant food when they can actually be a high glycemic food. Sweet potatoes have a glycemic index of 44 when boiled, but 94 when baked.

Whole Grains

Whole grains, such as brown rice and oatmeal, are permitted, as are products made with 100% whole grain flour. The authors explain that "wheat flour" is not whole grain flour. The ingredients list should state that flour is 100% whole wheat to be compliant. Grain products should also not contain added sugars.

Nuts and Legumes

Legumes (including many different types of beans) are a good source of protein and fiber and are lower in calories. They are an acceptable carbohydrate on this diet. Nuts and nut butters are also permitted, but read ingredient lists on nut butters closely and avoid those that contain added sugar.

Meats, Fish, and Eggs

The diet advises eating lean meats, removing the skin from poultry, and trimming the fat from lean beef, lamb. All fish and seafood are allowed, as are whole eggs. However, no breading is allowed on any meat or seafood products. Those on the Sugar Busters diet should also avoid meat cured in sugar (such as bacon and ham).

Low-Fat Dairy Products

Unsaturated fat is emphasized, but saturated fat is not forbidden. Butter is acceptable in moderation, for example, as are cream and cheese. Nonetheless, saturated fat should not comprise more than 10% of the diet. And low-fat dairy products should not contain added sugar.

High-Glycemic Fruits and Vegetables

High glycemic fruits and vegetables to avoid include bananas, raisins, pineapple, most root vegetables (white potatoes, beets, parsnips) as well as products made from those foods, like potato chips. Carrots are acceptable in moderation, as are 100% fruit juices that contain no added sugar.

Refined Carbohydrates

The diet has a list of refined carbohydrate foods that should be avoided, including white rice, white flour, and products made with white flour such as bread, cake, cookies, crackers, pretzels, doughnuts, bagels, and muffins. Whole grain pasta is allowed. Consumers may also want to consider legume pasta, as it includes more fiber and nutrients than refined pasta.

Sugar

Added sugar is off-limits. Honey, syrups, and products with added sugar are to be avoided. Readers are advised to avoid jams, jellies, some salad dressings, sauces (like ketchup and teriyaki sauce), soft drinks, and juice-based beverages that include added sugar.

Sample Shopping List

Shopping for foods on the Sugar Busters diet is pretty straightforward: avoid high GI foods (over 55) and balance your intake of protein, carbs, and fats according to your personalized plan. Steer clear of most packaged foods since they often contain added sugars and other artificial ingredients. In general, stick to real, whole foods whenever possible.

While what you eat on this plan is up to you, the following shopping list offers suggestions for getting started. Note this is not a definitive shopping list and there may be other foods that you prefer.

- Lean protein (chicken, lean beef, pork tenderloin, salmon, halibut, shrimp)

• Dark leafy greens (spinach, kale, Swiss chard, arugula)

• Veggies (broccoli, asparagus, celery, cucumber, peppers, spinach, tomatoes)

• Whole fruits (grapefruit, apple, peach, orange, grapes, cherries, strawberries)

• Whole grains (barley, brown rice, oat bran, whole-grain pasta, wheat tortillas)

• Legumes (black beans, lentils, chickpeas, kidney beans, split peas)

• Healthy fats (avocados, walnuts, almonds, pecans, olive oil)

• Low-fat dairy products (milk or dairy-free alternative, plain yogurt)

• Eggs

Health Benefits

Many people choose to follow low-carb and low-sugar diets to lose weight. In fact, a 2006 survey of more than 9,000 Americans following low-carb, high-protein diets (LCHP) like Sugar Busters, the Zone Diet, and Atkins showed a significant rate of weight loss among respondents, with 34% reporting an average loss of around 20 pounds. In addition, 40% of male and 30% of female respondents reported that they followed an LCHP diet long-term, which speaks to the sustainability of a low sugar lifestyle.

The health benefits of reducing your sugar intake are well-supported by scientific research and include a reduced risk for obesity, type 2 diabetes, and non-alcoholic fatty liver disease. A diet low in added sugars is also associated with improved heart health and reduced risk for metabolic syndrome and coronary disease.10 The basis of the Sugar Busters diet is about choosing low-glycemic foods to help regulate blood sugar, which is important for heart health, according to the American College of Cardiology.11

Health Risks

While there are no common health risks associated with the Sugar Busters diet, experts recommend approaching this plan with caution since the method eliminates healthy foods and lacks scientific evidence to justify these restrictions.

Additionally, restrictive eating plans without personalized guidelines can create unhealthy eating habits and nutritional imbalances. Since there is no calorie counting on the Sugar Busters diet, it's important to make sure you're still getting enough calories each day from a variety of nutrient-dense foods to maintain healthy blood sugar levels and balanced nutrition.

Sample Meal Plan

If you've relied on packaged or prepared foods, cooking your own meals from scratch may seem like a daunting process. But if you decide to follow the Sugar Busters diet and are adhering to its dietary restrictions, then you will likely spend more time in the kitchen cooking. Fortunately, there are many fresh and simple meals you can enjoy at home that are relatively easy to prepare.

The following three-day meal plan is not all-inclusive but should give you a general sense of what a few days on a well-balanced Sugar Busters diet could look like. You can accompany your meals with water, 100% fruit juice, or the occasional glass of dry red wine at dinner. Note that if you do choose to follow this program, there may be other meals that work better for you.

Day 1

Breakfast: vegetable omelet with peppers, onions, broccoli, and tomatoes

Lunch: grilled chicken with roasted asparagus and brown rice

Dinner: zucchini noodles with chicken meatballs and marinara sauce

Snacks: celery sticks with hummus, apple slices, and a handful of almonds

Day 2

Breakfast: almond milk smoothie with whey protein, spinach, and strawberries

Lunch: baked salmon with sweet potato wedges and a side salad

Dinner: Greek salad with grilled chicken, spinach, low-fat feta, tomatoes, olives, onions, cucumbers, and olive oil

Snacks: garlic roasted chickpeas, hard-boiled egg, and sliced pear

Day 3

Breakfast: oatmeal with cinnamon and plain, low-fat yogurt with berries

Lunch: stuffed bell pepper with turkey, quinoa, onions, tomatoes, garlic, and low-fat cheese

Dinner: stir-fry with beef, broccoli, peppers, cabbage, and onions

Snacks: kale chips, sliced peach, and low-fat cottage cheese

SUGAR BUSTERS DIET RECIPES

Trying new sugar buster-friendly recipes is a great way to explore new flavors and find new favorite dishes while looking after your health. In this part are nourishing sugar buster diet recipes for you to enjoy and lose weight fast.

Chicken with Pears and Blue Cheese

Preparation time

50 minutes

Ingredients

- 1 1/2 Tbsp whole grain pastry flour

- 1/2 tsp salt

- 1/4 tsp freshly ground black pepper

- 2 large boneless, skinless chicken breast halves (6–8 oz each), cut in half, or 4 chicken cutlets (3–4 oz each)

- 2 Tbsp canola oil

- 1 large onion, cut into wedges

- 2 medium pears, halved, cored, and sliced

- 1 bag (6 oz) baby spinach

- 1/2 c apple cider or apple juice

- 1 1/2 tsp fresh thyme leaves, or 1/2 tsp dried

- 1/2 c crumbled reduced-fat blue cheese

Instructions

1. Combine the flour, salt, and pepper in a shallow bowl.

2. Dredge the chicken in the mixture and set aside.

3. Heat 1 Tbsp of the oil in a large nonstick skillet over medium heat.

4. Add the onion and cook for 5 minutes, or until lightly browned.

5. Add the pears and cook for 3 minutes, or until lightly browned.

6. Add the spinach and cook for 1 minute, or until wilted.

7. Place mixture on a serving plate.

8. Heat the remaining 1 Tbsp oil in the same skillet.

9. Cook the chicken for 6 to 8 minutes, turning once, or until browned.

10. Add the cider and thyme and bring to a boil.

11. Reduce the heat to low and simmer for 5 minutes, or until the sauce is reduced by half.

12. Place the chicken on the spinach mixture, drizzle with the cider mixture, and sprinkle with the cheese.

Spiced Beef with Wasabi Cream

Preparation time

1 hour 20 minutes

Ingredients

- 1 tsp ground ginger

- 1 tsp Chinese five-spice powder

- 1/2 tsp garlic powder

- 1/2 tsp salt

- 1 beef eye round roast (about 2 lbs)

- 1 container (6 oz) fat-free Greek yogurt

- 1 tsp wasabi paste

- 4 heads baby bok choy, halved

- 6 oz shiitake mushrooms, stemmed and halved

- 1 red bell pepper, cut into strips

- 2 Tbsp canola oil

Instructions

1. Preheat the oven to 400°F.

2. In a small bowl, stir together the ginger, five-spice powder, garlic powder, and salt.

3. Place the beef on a baking sheet with sides.

4. Coat all sides of the beef with canola cooking spray.

5. Rub the ginger mixture over the beef. Bake for 15 minutes.

6. Reduce the heat to 350°F and bake for 50 to 60 minutes, or until a thermometer inserted in the center registers 145°F for medium rare, 160°F for medium, or 165°F for well done.

7. Remove to a serving plate and let stand for 15 minutes before carving.

8. Meanwhile, in a small bowl, stir together the yogurt and wasabi until smooth.

9. Cover and refrigerate until ready to serve.

10. Increase the oven temperature to 450°F while the roast stands.

11. Drain any liquid from the pan but leave some of the drippings.

12. Add the bok choy, mushrooms, pepper, and oil to the pan, tossing to coat.

13. Roast for 8 minutes, or until the vegetables are tender-crisp, stirring once.

14. Serve with 1/2 c hot cooked medium pearl barley per serving.

Stuffed Peppers Provence-Style

Preparation time

1 hour 20 minutes

Ingredients

- 4 medium bell peppers, any colors

- 1 navel orange

- 2 tsp olive oil

- 1 1/4 c finely chopped onion (1 large)

- 1 Tbsp minced garlic

- 1 tsp dried thyme

- 1 1/4 c no-salt-added small white beans, rinsed and drained

- 1/4 c fresh bread crumbs

- 2 Tbsp slivered Niçoise olives, or other ripe olives

- 2 Tbsp chopped parsley

- 1/4 tsp salt

- 1/4 tsp red-pepper flakes, extra for garnish

- 4 slices reduced-fat provolone cheese (such as Sargento), finely chopped

Instructions

1. Preheat the oven to 375°F. Coat a 13" x 9" microwave-safe baking dish with cooking spray.

2. Cut the peppers in half from stem to bottom.

3. Cut out and discard the ribs and seeds. Place the peppers, cut side down, in the dish.

4. Cover with plastic wrap, leaving a vent for steam to escape.

5. Microwave on high power for 5 minutes, or until hot and slightly softened.

6. Meanwhile, grate ½ tsp orange zest and set aside.

7. Squeeze 4 Tbsp orange juice and set aside.

8. Heat a nonstick skillet over medium heat.

9. Add the oil and heat for 1 minute.

10. Add the onion, garlic, and thyme.

11. Reduce the heat to low, cover, and cook, stirring occasionally, for 5 minutes, or until the onion starts to soften.

12. Add the beans, orange juice, and zest.

13. Partially cover the pan and simmer for 5 minutes.

14. Remove from the heat. Stir in the bread crumbs, olives, parsley, salt, and pepper flakes.

15. Allow to cool, stirring occasionally, for 10 minutes.

16. Turn the bell peppers cut side up in the baking dish.

17. Add all but 2 Tbsp of the cheese to the bean mixture and stir.

18.   Fill the peppers with the bean mixture, pressing down slightly.

19. Sprinkle on the remaining cheese.

20. Cover loosely with a sheet of foil.

21. Bake for about 30 minutes, or until the cheese is melted.

22. Allow to sit for 10 minutes before serving.

23. Pass additional pepper flakes at the table.

Autumn Chicken Stew in the Slow Cooker

Preparation time

8 hours 20 minutes

Ingredients

- 2 parsnips, peeled and cut into thirds

- 1 medium butternut squash, peeled, halved lengthwise, seeded, and cut into 1" slices

- 1 large red onion, cut into 8 wedges

- 1 c apple cider or apple juice

- 1 tsp dried rosemary

- 1 tsp dried thyme

- 1/2 tsp salt

- 4 boneless, skinless chicken breast halves (6 oz each)

- 6 oz baby spinach (about 6 c)

- 2 c cooked whole wheat couscous (2/3 cup dry)

Instructions

1. Arrange the parsnips, squash, and onion in a 4- or 5-quart slow cooker.

2. Pour the cider over the vegetables and sprinkle with 1/2 tsp of the rosemary, 1/2 tsp of the thyme, and 1/4 tsp of the salt.

3. Lay the chicken on the vegetables and sprinkle with the remaining 1/2 tsp rosemary, 1/2 tsp thyme, and 1/4 tsp salt.

4. Cover and cook on low for 6 to 8 hours. Stir the spinach into the hot liquid until wilted.

5. Divide the vegetables into 4 soup bowls.

6. Top each with a chicken breast half and some sauce.

7. Top each bowl with 1/2 c of the hot couscous.

Seared Caribbean Scallops with Black Bean Salsa

Preparation time

45 minutes

Ingredients

- 1 tsp Caribbean jerk seasoning

- 12 sea scallops (1 oz each), preferably dry caught

- 2 Tbsp canola oil

- 1 can (14 1/2 oz) no-salt-added black beans, rinsed and drained

- 1 medium tomato, chopped

- 3/4 c chopped red bell pepper (about 1 medium)

- 1/2 medium red onion, finely chopped

- 1 small jalapeño pepper, finely chopped (wear plastic gloves when handling)

- 1 c cubed mango

- 1/4 tsp ground cumin

- 1 Tbsp chopped cilantro

- 2 Tbsp lime juice

- 4 lime wedges

- 1/8 tsp salt

- freshly ground black pepper

Instructions

1. Place the scallops on a work surface.

2. Pat dry.

3. Dust with the jerk seasoning and toss to coat evenly.

4. Set aside.

5. In a medium bowl, combine the beans, tomato, bell pepper, onion, jalapeño pepper,

mango, cumin, cilantro, lime juice, 1 Tbsp of the canola oil, and salt and pepper to taste.

6. Mix well to combine.

7. Let stand to blend flavors.

8. Meanwhile, heat a skillet over medium-high heat.

9. Add the remaining 1 Tbsp of canola oil and heat for 1 minute.

10. Add the scallops to the skillet.

11. Cook for 1 to 2 minutes on each side, 2 to 4 minutes total, until well browned all over and opaque in the center.

12. Remove to a plate.

13. Spoon the salsa onto 4 dinner plates.

14. Top with the scallops.

15. Place a lime wedge on each plate.

Pasta Primavera

Preparation time

31 minutes

Ingredients

- 2 Tbsp canola oil

- 1 clove garlic, chopped

- 1 c thinly sliced carrots (2 medium)

- 1 c thinly sliced onions (1 medium)

- 1 c frozen baby peas, rinsed and drained

- 1 c frozen artichoke hearts, thawed

- 1/4 c reduced-sodium vegetable broth

- 6 oz whole wheat spaghetti

- 1/2 c slivered fresh basil

- 1/4 c grated Parmesan or romano cheese

- freshly ground black pepper

Instructions

1. Prepare the pasta according to package directions for al dente.

2. Reserve ½ c of the cooking water before draining.

3. Heat the oil in a deep, wide, nonstick skillet over medium-high heat for 1 minute.

4. Add the garlic, carrots, and onions. Cook, stirring frequently, for 5 minutes, or until the vegetables start to soften.

5. Add the peas and artichokes.

6. Cook, stirring frequently, for 2 minutes, just until heated.

7. Add the broth.

8. Keep warm over low heat.

9. Add the pasta and the basil to the skillet and toss to combine. Add some of the reserved pasta water to moisten if necessary.

10.   Allow to sit for 1 minute so flavors will blend.

11. Add the cheese and toss.

12. Serve immediately.

13. Season with pepper at the table.

Pan-Grilled Mediterranean Salmon

Preparation time

32 minutes

Ingredients

- 3/4 cup chopped red onion (1/2- 3/4 medium)

- 1 tablespoon minced garlic (2-3 large cloves)

- 2 teaspoons crumbled dried sage

- 2 teaspoons canola oil

- 1 can (15 1/2 ounces) no-salt-added cannellini beans, rinsed and drained

- 1/2 cup fat-free, reduced-sodium chicken broth

- 1/4 teaspoon salt

- 3 cups baby spinach

- 2 teaspoons flaxseed oil

- 4 skinless salmon fillets (3 ounces each)

- red-pepper flakes

Instructions

1. Combine the onion, garlic, 1 1/2 teaspoons sage, and oil in a deep, wide skillet.

2. Cover and cook over medium heat, stirring occasionally, for about 5 minutes or until the onion starts to soften.

3. Add the beans, broth, and salt. Simmer for about 10 minutes.

4. Stir the spinach into the beans and cook for another 2 to 3 minutes.

5. Stir the flaxseed oil into the bean mixture.

6. Remove the pan from the heat.

7. Rub the salmon fillets with the remaining sage.

8. Heat the remaining oil in a medium skillet or grill pan.

9. Place the salmon fillets in the pan and cook for 3 to 4 minutes.

10. Carefully turn each fillet and cook for 1 minute longer.

11. Remove the fillets to 4 plates.

12. Spoon the beans onto each plate.

13. Serve with the pepper flakes.

Parmesan Chicken Strips with Garlicky Escarole and Fennel

Preparation time

35 minutes

Ingredients

- 1/2 c white panko breadcrumbs

- 1/2 c shredded Parmesan cheese

- 1/4 tsp freshly ground black pepper

- 1 omega-3-enriched egg

- 2 Tbsp water

- 4 boneless, skinless chicken breast halves, cut into 1" slices

- 2 Tbsp canola oil

- 1 large head fennel, cut into thin wedges

- 1 red onion, cut into thin wedges

- 2 cloves garlic, minced

- 10–12 c escarole, cut into thin strips (about 1 large head)

Instructions

1. Preheat the oven to 400°F.

2. Coat a large baking sheet with cooking spray.

3. On a plate, combine the panko, cheese, and pepper.

4. In a shallow bowl, combine the egg and water and beat with a fork.

5. Dip the chicken, a few strips at a time, into the egg mixture and then into the panko mixture, pressing to coat well.

6. Place on the baking sheet and coat top of chicken with cooking spray.

7. Bake, turning once, for 10 minutes, or until a thermometer inserted in the center reaches 160ºF.

8. Meanwhile, heat the oil in a large skillet over medium-high heat. Add the fennel and onion, reduce the heat to medium, and cook for 4 minutes, or until browned.

9. Add the garlic and cook for 1 minute. Stir in the escarole and cook for 4 minutes, or until wilted.

10. Divide the escarole mixture onto 4 plates.

11. Top with the chicken strips.

Curried Lentils and Cauliflower

Preparation time

55 minutes

Ingredients

- 3 tsp canola oil

- 4 c cauliflower florets, cut into small pieces (12–16 oz)

- 1/2 c chopped onion (1 small)

- 1/2 c chopped carrot (1 medium)

- 1 c dried brown lentils

- 2 tsp minced garlic

- 1 tsp curry powder

- 1 1/2 c reduced-sodium vegetable broth

- 1/4 tsp salt

- 1/2 c fat-free plain yogurt

- fresh cilantro leaves

Instructions

1. Heat a large, deep skillet over medium-high heat.

2. Add 2 tsp of the oil. Heat for 1 minute.

3. Add the cauliflower.

4. Cover and cook, tossing occasionally, for 5 minutes, or until the cauliflower is lightly charred.

5. Reduce the heat if the cauliflower is browning too quickly.

6. Remove the cauliflower to a plate. Set aside.

7. Return the skillet to medium heat.

8. Add the remaining 1 tsp of oil and the onion and carrot.

9. Cook, stirring, for 3 minutes, or until the vegetables start to soften.

10. Stir in the lentils, garlic, and curry powder.

11. Cook, stirring, for 3 minutes to coat the lentils with the seasonings.

12. Add the broth.

13. Bring almost to a boil.

14. Partially cover the pan and reduce the heat.

15. Simmer for about 20 minutes, or until the lentils are almost tender.

16. Add the cauliflower to the skillet.

17. Partially cover and simmer for about 5 minutes, or until the cauliflower is tender and the lentils are cooked.

18. Stir in the salt

19. Spoon into 4 pasta bowls.

20. Divide and dollop on the yogurt.

21. Garnish with cilantro.

Chicken Roll-Ups

Preparation time

29 minutes

Ingredients

- 2 Tbsp hoisin sauce

- 2 Tbsp rice wine vinegar

- 1 Tbsp reduced-sodium soy sauce

- 1 tsp toasted sesame oil

- 1 lb boneless, skinless chicken breasts, cut into ¼" cubes

- 4 scallions, chopped

- 2 carrots, shredded (about 1½ c)

- 1 clove garlic, minced

- 1 Tbsp finely chopped ginger

- ¼ c water

- 2 oz walnuts, toasted and coarsely chopped (½ c)

- 1 c sliced canned water chestnuts

- 12 Bibb or Boston lettuce leaves

Instructions

1. In a medium bowl, stir together the hoisin, vinegar, soy sauce, and oil. Stir in the chicken, tossing to coat.

2. Let stand 10 minutes.

3. Heat a nonstick skillet coated with cooking spray over medium heat.

4. Remove the chicken from the marinade with a slotted spoon.

5. Reserve the marinade. Cook chicken for 5 minutes, stirring, until browned.

6. Add the scallions, carrots, garlic, and ginger and cook for 3 minutes, or until tender.

7. Stir in the reserved marinade and the water.

8. Cook, bringing to a boil and stirring constantly, for 1 to 2 minutes, or until thickened.

9. Stir in the walnuts and water chestnuts.

10. Place 3 lettuce leaves on each of 4 plates and fill with ¼ c of the chicken mixture.

Penne with Pepper Steak and Caramelized Onions

Preparation time

1 hour 20 minutes

Ingredients

- 3/4 lb flank steak

- 2 Tbsp cracked black pepper

- 2 cloves garlic, minced

- 1 Tbsp canola oil

- 1 large yellow onion, sliced

- 1 red onion, sliced

- 2 Tbsp balsamic vinegar

- 1 c reduced-sodium beef broth

- 8 oz penne pasta (such as Barilla Plus)

- 6 oz baby arugula

- shaved Parmesan cheese

Instructions

1. Preheat the broiler.

2. Place the flank steak on the rack of a broiler pan and coat all sides with the pepper and garlic.

3. Let stand about 10 minutes.

4. Heat the oil in a large skillet over medium-high heat.

5. Cook the onions for 8 minutes, or until lightly browned.

6. Reduce the heat to medium-low and add the vinegar to deglaze.

7. Stir in the broth, cover, and cook for 15 minutes, or until the onions are very soft and browned.

8. Remove from the heat.

9. Prepare the pasta according to package directions, drain, and place in a large bowl.

10. Meanwhile, broil the steak, 4 inches from the heat, for 12 minutes, or until a thermometer inserted in the center registers 145°F for medium rare, 160°F for medium, or 165°F for well done.

11. Let stand for 10 minutes, then slice into thin strips.

12. Stir the arugula into the onions.

13. Add the pasta and toss to coat.

14. Add the steak strips and top with the cheese.

Lemon-Pepper Crusted Halibut with Butternut Squash Puree

Preparation time

40 minutes

Ingredients

- 1 slice whole wheat bread

- 1 container (20 oz) peeled butternut squash

- 3 large cloves garlic, unpeeled

- 1 Tbsp ground flaxseed

- 1 tsp lemon-pepper seasoning

- 1/4 tsp salt

- 2 Tbsp white whole wheat flour (such as King Arthur)

- 1 omega-3-enriched egg white

- 1 Tbsp water

- 4 boneless halibut fillets (3 oz each)

- 1 Tbsp canola oil

- 2 Tbsp nonfat dry milk

- 1 Tbsp chopped parsley

Instructions

1. Preheat the oven to 375°F.

2. Line a baking sheet with foil.

3. Coat the foil with cooking spray.

4. Toast the bread until it is very crisp.

5. Set it aside to cool.

6. Place the squash and garlic in a single layer on a microwave-safe dish.

7. Cover with plastic wrap, leaving a vent.

8. Microwave on high power, rotating occasionally, for about 10 minutes, or until very soft.

9. Remove and set aside.

10. Meanwhile, break the toast into small chunks. Place in the bowl of a food processor fitted with a metal blade.

11. Process for about 2 minutes, or until fine crumbs form. Measure out 3 Tbsp and place on a large sheet of waxed paper. (Freeze the remaining crumbs for another recipe.)

12. Add the flaxseed, seasoning, and 1/8 tsp of the salt. Using clean hands, mix with your fingers.

13. Place the flour on a second sheet of waxed paper.

14. In a shallow bowl, combine the egg white and water and beat with a fork.

15. One at a time, dip each fish fillet into the flour to coat it.

16. Shake off the excess. (Not all of the flour will be used.)

17. Dip the fish into the egg mixture, shaking off the excess.

18. Dip the fish into the flaxseed mixture to coat evenly.

19. Place on the prepared baking sheet.

20. Press any remaining flaxseed mixture evenly on top of the fish.

21. Drizzle evenly with the oil.

22. Bake for 10 minutes, or until opaque in the center.

23. Meanwhile, transfer the squash to the bowl of a food processor fitted with a metal blade.

24. Pop the garlic from its skin and add it to the bowl along with the dry milk and the remaining 1/8 tsp salt.

25. Process, scraping the bowl as needed, for about 2 minutes, or until smooth.

26. Divide the squash onto 4 dinner plates.

27. Top each with a fish fillet.

28. Sprinkle on the parsley.

Paleo Sweet Potato Blueberry Breakfast Bars

Preparation time

50 minutes

Ingredients

- 3/4 cup mashed sweet potato

- 1 tablespoon vanilla extract

- 1 tablespoon coconut oil, melted

- 1 tablespoon raw honey

- 1 egg

- 1/2 cup almond meal

- 1/8 cup coconut flour

- 3/4 teaspoon baking powder

- 1/2 cup blueberries

Instructions

1. Preheat oven to 350 degrees

2. Roast or microwave one large sweet potato until soft.

3. Scoop out the inside and reserve 3/4 cup

4. In a medium bowl, combine the mashed sweet potato, vanilla extract, melted coconut oil, raw honey, and egg

5. Add the almond meal, coconut flour, and baking powder.

6. Mix well

7. Grease a 9×5 inch loaf pan and pour in the batter, pushing it into all the corners and middle of the pan to avoid large air bubbles.

8. Smooth out the top

9. Place the blueberries in a single layer on the top and gently press the berries into the batter

10. Bake for 35-40 minutes, or until the middle is set

11. Let cool and cut into small bars.

12. Serve immediately or refrigerate to store

RANCH KALE CHIPS

Preparation time

30 minutes

Ingredients

- 1 bunch lacinato kale

- 3 tablespoons olive oil

• 2–3 teaspoons Hidden Valley® Original Ranch® Seasoning, Salad Dressing & Recipe Mix Packet

Instructions

1. Preheat oven to 275°F.

2. Wash and dry the kale thoroughly, and remove the tough inner ribs from each leaf.

3. Cut into bite-size pieces.

4. In a bowl, toss the leaves with the oil and Salad Dressing & Seasoning mix, using your hands to massage the seasoning into the leaves.

5. Spread leaves in one layer on two lightly greased baking sheets.

6.   Place in oven and bake until crisped and starting to brown on the edges, about 20–25 minutes.

7. About halfway through cooking time, remove tray, shake or redistribute leaves with a spatula, and switch the positions of the trays in the oven. If some of the leaves start to get brown and crisp before the others, it's OK to remove and place the unfinished ones back in the oven.

Tip:

1. Get the lacinato (also called Dino or Tuscan) kale for this recipe, as the leaves hold up best. If you can't find that, it's fine to substitute curly kale.

2. Some heads are bigger than others, so you may need to adjust the amount of oil and seasoning, as indicated below.

CHOCOLATE PEANUT BUTTER MUFFINS

Preparation time

25 minutes

INGREDIENTS

- 2 eggs

- 1/2 cup peanut butter

- 1/2 cup 2% fat cottage cheese

- 1 teaspoon vanilla

- 1 teaspoon baking soda

- 1 tablespoon cocoa powder

- 8 -10g artificial sweetener

Instructions

1. Preheat oven to 350.

2. Line a cup cake pan with paper cups.

3. Microwave the peanut butter for 45 seconds to melt.

4. Add everything to a medium sized bowl and mix well. 1 packet of artificial sweetener = 1 gram.

5. Spoon into 9 cup cake cups and bake for 15 minutes.

Banana, apple and blueberry loaf

Preparation time

1 hour 15 minutes

INGREDIENTS

- 1 vanilla bean, seeds scraped

- 225g unsalted butter, softened

- 1 cup (140g) coconut sugar

- 2 ripe bananas, flesh mashed with a fork

- 3 eggs

- 2 apples, 1 grated, 1 thinly sliced

- 125g blueberries, crushed with a fork

- ½ cup (100g) rice flour

- 3/4 cup (85g) coconut flour

- 1 3/4 cup (175g) almond meal

- 1/2 tsp bicarbonate of soda

- 1/2 tsp baking powder

- 1/4 cup (60ml) almond milk

- 1/4 cup (90g) honey, plus extra to drizzle

SPICE POWDER

- 2 whole star anise

- 1 tsp white peppercorns

- 2 small cinnamon quills

- 1/2 tsp cloves

- Seeds from 2 tsp cardamom pods

- 2 tsp juniper berries (optional)

- 1 pinch saffron threads

- 1 tsp Murray River sea salt flakes

Instructions

1. Preheat oven to 180°C.

2. For spice powder, place star anise, peppercorns, cinnamon, cloves and cardamom in a pan over medium heat and cook 1-2 minutes until fragrant.

3. Place in mortar and pestle with the juniper berries, saffron and salt.

4. Crush to a powder.

5. In a stand mixer, beat vanilla, 200g butter and sugar.

6. Add banana and eggs, one at a time. On low, add 1½ tsp spice powder, grated apple, blueberries, flours, almond meal, baking powder, bicarb, 1 tsp salt and almond milk.

7. Beat until well combined.

8. Pour into a greased 24x12cm loaf tin.

9. Bake 1 hour 15 minutes or until skewer comes out clean.

10. Put 25g butter and honey in a frypan over medium heat.

11. Add apple slices.

12. Cook 3-4 minutes, turning, until carmelised.

13. Place on top of bread.

14. Serve drizzled with honey.

Berry's antioxidant happiness smoothie

Preparation time

15 minutes

INGREDIENTS

- 2 cups frozen blueberries

- 2 tablespoons maple syrup

• 1–2 cups almond milk

TO SERVE

• Fresh blueberries, whole or halved

• Granola

Instructions

1. Pop everything into a blender and whizz it all up to your preferred consistency.

2. To serve, cover the bottom of two glasses with a few fresh blueberries and a little paleo granola, then fill them up with the smoothie and top with more blueberries and granola. This way you've got the prettiness at the top of your smoothie and the surprise at the bottom too!

Eggs poached in spicy tomato sauce

Preparation time

25 minutes

INGREDIENTS

- ¼ cup (60ml) extra virgin olive oil

- 2 eschalots, finely chopped

- 1 celery stick, finely chopped

- ½ bunch flat-leaf parsley, stalks and leaves chopped

- 2 garlic cloves, chopped

- 1 long red chilli, finely chopped, plus extra slices to serve

- 700g jar of passata

- 4 eggs

- Crusty bread to serve

Instructions

1. Heat the olive oil in a saucepan over medium heat.

2. Add the eschalots, celery, parsley stalks, garlic and chilli and cook for 2-3 minutes until the eschalots are translucent and golden.

3. Add the passata and ½ cup (125ml) water and bring to the boil.

4. Reduce the heat to low and simmer gently for 15 minutes.

5. Make small holes in the pan with your spoon then crack the eggs in one by one.

6. Cook for 5-6 minutes until the whites are set but the yolks are still runny.

7. Remove from the heat, top with parsley leaves and extra chilli and serve hot with crusty bread.

Raw vegies, ricotta, eggs and green sauce

Preparation time

20 minutes

INGREDIENTS

- 1 cup (200g) buckwheat

- 1 bunch mixed radishes, trimmed, halved (reserve leaves for salsa verde)

- 1 bunch baby (Dutch) carrots, trimmed, peeled (reserve leaves for salsa verde)

- 2 tbs apple cider vinegar

- 2 slices dark rye bread, torn

- 1/4 cup (60ml) olive oil

- 4 eggs, at room temperature

- 500g fresh ricotta, cut into 4 wedges

- 2 Lebanese cucumbers, thinly sliced

- 150g heirloom cherry tomatoes, halved

- 1 cup loosely packed watercress sprigs

CARROT AND RADISH LEAF SALSA VERDE

- 1/2 cup loosely packed reserved carrot and radish leaves

- 1 pickled gherkin, chopped

- 1 cup loosely packed flat-leaf parsley leaves

- 1/4 cup loosely packed dill fronds

- 1 garlic clove, chopped

- 1 tbs Dijon mustard

- 1/4 cup (60ml) apple cider vinegar

- 1 tbs baby capers, drained

- 2 tsp honey

- 1/3 cup (80ml) olive oil

Instructions

1. Cook buckwheat in a saucepan of boiling salted water for 9 minutes or until tender.

2. Refresh, drain and set aside.

3. Toss radish and carrot in a bowl with vinegar and 1 tsp salt flakes. Chill for at least 30 minutes

to pickle. (Pickled vegetables can be stored, covered and chilled, for up to 2 days.)

4. Meanwhile, for the salsa verde, place all ingredients in a food processor and whiz to a smooth paste.

5. Transfer to a bowl and cover surface with plastic wrap until required. (Salsa verde can be stored, covered and chilled, for up to 1 week.)

6. Wipe food processor clean.

7. Add bread and whiz to fine crumbs. Heat oil in a frypan over medium-high heat.

8. Add breadcrumbs and cook, stirring, for 3 minutes or until crisp.

9. Remove and drain on paper towel.

10. Cook eggs in a saucepan of boiling water for 6 1/2 minutes.

11. Transfer to a bowl of iced water and peel when cool enough to handle.

12. Divide buckwheat and ricotta among serving bowls.

13. Top with cucumber, tomato, drained pickled vegetables, halved eggs and watercress.

14. Scatter with breadcrumbs, drizzle with a little salsa verde and serve with remaining salsa verde on the side.

Egg, bacon and tomato tart

Preparation time

35 minutes

INGREDIENTS

- 200g sour cream or creme fraiche

- 2 tsp chopped thyme leaves, plus extra to serve

- 2 tsp Dijon mustard

- 150g cherry tomatoes, halved

- 2 truss tomatoes, cut into wedges

- 6 smoky bacon rashers

- 6 eggs

- 2 tbs pure (thin) cream

- 2 tbs finely grated cheddar cheese

CHEDDAR PASTRY

- 125g each plain and wholemeal flour

- 150g chilled unsalted butter, cut into small pieces

- 100g cheddar cheese, coarsely grated

- 1 egg

- 1 tbs white vinegar

Instructions

1. For the cheddar pastry, combine the flours, butter, cheddar and a pinch of salt in a food processor and pulse until combined, but still with small lumps of butter.

2. Tip onto a work surface and make a well in the centre.

3. Combine the egg and vinegar in a bowl, mixing with a fork, then add to the well, gently incorporating into the dry ingredients until a rough dough forms.

4. Lightly knead to form into a disc, wrap in plastic wrap and refrigerate to rest for 1 hour.

5. Roll out pastry on a lightly floured surface to a rough 30x40cm rectangle and line a 20x30cm baking tray, pressing into the corners.

6. Trim so the edges overhang sides by about 2cm.

7. Refrigerate until required.

8. Preheat the oven to 180°C.

9. Combine sour cream, thyme and mustard in a bowl, spread over base of the tart, then scatter tomatoes over the top, leaving six gaps (these gaps are where the eggs will fit).

10. Tear the bacon into rough pieces and tuck around the tomatoes, then carefully crack an egg into each gap, being careful not to break the yolks.

11. Drizzle over the cream, scatter with the cheddar and season, then gently fold in the overhanging pastry to form a rough border.

12. Bake for 30-35 minutes until the pastry is golden brown and the eggs are set.

13. Serve the tart warm or at room temperature, scattered with extra thyme.

Spicy chickpeas with soppressata and eggs

Preparation time

30 minutes

INGREDIENTS

- 2 tbs extra virgin olive oil

- 2 eschalots, thinly sliced

- 1 tbs finely chopped flat-leaf parsley stalks

- 1 small green chilli, thinly sliced

- 1 garlic clove, crushed

- 100g soppressata (Italian dry salami), cut into 2cm pieces

- 2 x 400g cans chickpeas, rinsed, drained

- 1/2 cup (125ml) tomato passata (sugo)

- 4 eggs

Instructions

1. Heat oil in a large, heavy-based frypan over medium heat.

2. Add eschalot, parsley stalks, chilli, garlic and soppressata, and cook, stirring, for 2-3 minutes until eschalot begins to soften.

3. Add chickpeas and cook, stirring to coat, for a further 1-2 minutes.

4. Add passata and 1 cup (250ml) water, then reduce heat to low.

5. Cook for 10-15 minutes until slightly reduced.

6. Season.

7. Make 4 small indents in the mixture and crack an egg into each.

8. Cook for 3-4 minutes until whites are cooked. Serve immediately.

Vegan banana bread

Preparation time

1 hour

INGREDIENTS

• 450g mashed banana (about 5-6 bananas), plus 2 extra sliced bananas

• 1/4 cup (60ml) maple syrup

• 1/4 cup (60ml) extra virgin olive oil or macadamia oil

• 1 tsp ground cinnamon

• 2 tsp baking powder

- 2 cups (180g) desiccated coconut

- 1 3/4 cup (175g) almond meal

- 1/3 cup (25g) shredded coconut

Instructions

1. Preheat oven to 180°C. Grease the base and sides of a 1.5L-capacity loaf pan and line with baking paper.

2. Combine mashed banana, maple syrup, oil, cinnamon and baking powder in a bowl.

3. Add the desiccated coconut and almond meal, and combine well.

4. Spoon into prepared pan and top with sliced banana and shredded coconut.

5. Bake for 1 hour or until a skewer inserted in the centre comes out clean.

6. Cool completely in pan before serving.

Italian sausage and fennel tartlets with quail eggs

Preparation time

1 hour 30 minutes

INGREDIENTS

- 3 sheets frozen shortcrust pastry, thawed

- 2 tablespoons olive oil

- 200g Italian pork and fennel sausages, casings removed

- 100g bacon, finely chopped

- 1/2 teaspoon ground fennel

- 1 tablespoon finely chopped tarragon leaves

- 1/2 teaspoon dried chilli flakes

- 2 tablespoons sour cream

- 50g semi-dried tomatoes, finely chopped

- 24 quail eggs (see note)

- 6 pickled jalapenos, drained, sliced

- Thyme leaves, to serve

Instructions

1. Preheat the oven to 180°C. Lightly grease two 12-hole muffin pans.

2. Cut 24 x 8cm pastry circles, then use to line the muffin pans.

3. Line each pastry case with baking paper and baking weights or uncooked rice and bake for 20 minutes or until golden and almost dry.

4. Remove weights and paper and cool.

5. Meanwhile, place oil in a large, non-stick frypan over medium heat.

6. Cook sausage meat and bacon for 8-10 minutes, breaking up any lumps with a wooden spoon, until golden and cooked through.

7. Add the fennel, tarragon and chilli flakes, then season with salt and freshly ground black pepper.

8. Cook, stirring, for a further 2-3 minutes until fragrant, then stir in sour cream and semi-dried tomato.

9. Fill each pastry case with 1/2 teaspoon sausage mixture.

10. Carefully crack a quail egg on top, then top each tartlet with a few thin slices of jalapeno and season.

11. Bake tartlets for 15-20 minutes or until the eggs are set.

12. Sprinkle the tartlets with thyme leaves and serve warm.

Shanghai breakfast pancake

Preparation time

40 minutes

INGREDIENTS

• Sunflower oil, to deep-fry

• 6 wonton wrappers

• 6 free-range eggs

• 2 tbs hoisin sauce, plus extra to serve (optional)

• 1 long red chilli, seeds removed, chopped

• 3 spring onions, thinly sliced

CREPES

- 1 cup (150g) plain flour

- 300ml milk

- 1 large (70g) egg

- 40g unsalted butter, melted,

- plus extra to brush (or use oil spray)

Instructions

1. For the crepes, whiz the flour, milk and egg in a food processor or blender until smooth.

2. Add the butter, then process to combine.

3. Transfer to a jug, then cover and stand for 30 minutes at room temperature.

4. Meanwhile, half-fill a small saucepan or deep-fryer with sunflower oil and heat to 180°C (a cube of bread will turn golden in 30 seconds when the oil is hot enough).

5. Fry wonton wrappers, one at a time, for 30 seconds (turning once) until crisp, then carefully remove with tongs or a slotted spoon and drain on paper towel.

6. When cool enough to handle, break into large pieces.

7. Heat a 20cm non-stick frypan or crepe pan over medium heat.

8. Lightly grease pan with melted butter or oil spray.

9. Pour 50ml (2 1/2 tablespoons) crepe mixture in the pan, tilting to coat the base.

10. Cook for 1 minute or until golden, then flip the crepe over.

11. Crack an egg onto the crepe, then use a spatula to gently break up the egg and smear it over the surface of the crepe.

12. Sprinkle with some spring onion and fried wonton wrapper.

13. Fold the crepe in half, then smear 1 teaspoon hoisin over the top and sprinkle with some of the chilli. Finally, fold in half again to form a triangle.

14. Remove from the frypan and keep warm while you make remaining pancakes.

15. Just before serving, drizzle with extra hoisin, if desired, and top with extra spring onion.

Broccolini, pea and asparagus breakfast gratin

Preparation time

20 minutes

INGREDIENTS

- 100g speck, finely chopped

- 2 bunches broccolini, stalks sliced, florets reserved

- 3 cups (480g) fresh peas, blanched, refreshed in iced water

- 2 bunches asparagus, thinly sliced lengthways

- 150g baby spinach leaves

- 1 tsp dried chilli flakes

- 1 1/2 tbs extra virgin olive oil

- 400g ricotta, broken into large chunks

- 2 cups (220g) grated mozzarella

- 6 eggs, poached

- Micro or flat-leaf parsley, to serve

Instructions

1. Preheat grill to high.

2.   Place speck in a cold non-stick frypan and place over medium heat. Cook, stirring, for 5 minutes or until golden and crisp.

3. Add broccolini stalks and cook, stirring, for 1-2 minutes until tender.

4. Add broccolini florets, peas, asparagus and spinach, and cook for a further 1 minute or until spinach is just wilted.

5. Transfer to a bowl and toss with chilli flakes and oil, then season.

6. Stir through ricotta and half of the mozzarella.

7. Divide the mixture among six 400ml-capacity ovenproof gratin dishes, then scatter over remaining mozzarella.

8. Grill for 8 minutes or until golden and bubbling.

9. Serve each topped with a poached egg and parsley.

Dukkah eggs

Preparation time

10 minutes

INGREDIENTS

• 6 hard-boiled eggs

• 1 tablespoon olive oil

• 2 cups dukkah

- 1 tablespoon harissa paste, or to taste

- 1 cup (280g) thick Greek yoghurt

Instructions

1. Peel the eggs and brush with the olive oil.

2. Roll the eggs in the dukkah.

3. To serve, swirl the harissa through the yoghurt.

4. Quarter the eggs and serve with the yoghurt for dipping.

Zucchini fritters with smoked salmon and poached eggs

Preparation time

40 minutes

INGREDIENTS

- 300g zucchinis, coarsely grated

- 1 small onion, finely chopped

- 2 garlic cloves, finely chopped

- 3/4 cup flat-leaf parsley leaves, chopped

- 1/2 cup mint leaves, chopped

- 1/2 cup dill sprigs, chopped, plus extra sprigs to serve

- 10 eggs, 2 lightly beaten, 8 poached

- 1/4 cup (40g) plain wholemeal flour

- 50g goat's cheese, broken into chunks

- 50g ricotta

- 2 tbs olive oil

- 8 large slices smoked salmon

Instructions

1. Place zucchini in a bowl and sprinkle with 1 tsp salt.

2. Combine well and set aside for 30 minutes, then strain off excess liquid and discard.

3. Return the zucchini to the bowl with the onion, garlic, parsley, mint, dill and 2 beaten eggs, and combine well.

4. Add the flour and stir to combine.

5. Fold in the goat's cheese and ricotta without overmixing – it's nice to have big chunks.

6. Heat 1 tbs oil in a large non-stick frypan over medium heat.

7. Using 1/4 cup (60ml) batter for each fritter, add 4 fritters to pan and cook for 2 minutes or until golden.

8. Flip and cook for a further 2 minutes or until cooked through.

9. Repeat with remaining oil and batter. (If you like crispier fritters, place in a preheated 180°C oven for an extra 5 minutes after frying.)

10. Serve fritters layered with salmon and topped with the poached eggs.

11. Garnish with the extra dill sprigs.

Soft-boiled eggs with dippers

Preparation time

12 minutes

INGREDIENTS

• 6 eggs, brought to room temperature

• Toast soldiers, to dip

- Roasted cherry tomatoes, to dip

- Carrot sticks, to dip

- Fried pancetta, to dip

- Roast vegetable chips, to dip

Instructions

1. Place eggs in a saucepan, cover with cold water and bring to the boil.

2. Reduce heat to medium and simmer for 3 minutes for soft-boiled.

3. Transfer eggs to egg cups, remove the tops, then serve with dippers.